# Banana Pineapple Drink That Melt Fat Like Crazy: Slimming Tropical Fusion, Banana Pineapple Fat-Burner.

Dr. Robert Anderson

# Copy Right

# Introduction

Welcome to 'Banana Pineapple Drink That Burns Fat Like Crazy'! In this low-content book, you'll discover the delicious and effective secrets to turbocharge your fat-burning journey. Get ready to sip your way to a healthier, slimmer you with mouthwatering recipes and insightful tips. Let's embark on this flavorful adventure together!"

# Table Of Contents

# Chapter 1

## Introduction to the Fat-Melting Power of Banana Pineapple Drink

*Welcome to the world of fat-burning beverages, where the fusion of two tropical powerhouses—banana and pineapple—creates a potent elixir that ignites your body's natural fat-burning mechanisms.*
*In this chapter, we embark on a journey to uncover the miraculous properties of these fruits and their synergistic effects when blended into a delicious and refreshing drink.*

*Bananas, with their rich reserves of potassium, fibre, and essential vitamins, have long been hailed as a nutritional powerhouse. They provide sustained energy, regulate digestion, and support muscle function—all vital components of a healthy metabolism. Pineapples, on the other hand, boast an impressive enzyme called bromelain, known for its ability to aid digestion, reduce inflammation, and accelerate the breakdown of fats.*

*When these two super-fruits are combined, their individual benefits amplify, creating a beverage that not only tantalises the taste buds but also revs up the body's fat-burning furnace. But how exactly does this magical elixir work its slimming wonders?*

*The secret lies in the unique combination of nutrients found in bananas and pineapples. Potassium and fibre from bananas help regulate fluid balance and curb cravings, while bromelain from pineapples enhances digestion and nutrient absorption. Together, they form a dynamic duo that targets stubborn fat stores, kickstarting your metabolism into high gear. Throughout this book, we'll delve deeper into the science behind the fat-melting power of banana pineapple drink, exploring its effects on metabolism, appetite control, and overall well-being. Whether you're looking to shed a few pounds or simply boost your energy levels, this tropical concoction offers a delicious and effective solution.*

*So, grab your blender and prepare to embark on a journey to a healthier, slimmer you. With each sip of banana pineapple drink, you're not only treating your taste buds to a burst of tropical flavour but also fueling your body with the nutrients it needs to torch fat and thrive. Get ready to experience the transformative power of nature's own fat-burning elixir.*

# Chapter 2

## Understanding the Ingredients.

*In our quest to unlock the secrets of the "Banana Pineapple Drink that Burns Fat Like Crazy," it's crucial to delve into the nutritional powerhouse that forms its foundation: bananas and pineapples.*

### *Bananas:*

*Bananas, often hailed as nature's perfect snack, are packed with essential nutrients that contribute to overall well-being. Rich in dietary fibre, bananas aid in digestion by promoting regular bowel movements and preventing constipation. This fibre content also helps to keep you feeling full for longer periods, reducing the likelihood of overeating and supporting weight management efforts.*

*Beyond fibre, bananas boast an impressive array of vitamins and minerals. They are particularly high in potassium, a vital electrolyte that plays a crucial role in maintaining fluid balance, muscle function, and heart health. Additionally, bananas contain significant levels of vitamin C, vitamin B6, and manganese, all of which contribute to immune function, energy metabolism, and antioxidant defence.*

### *Pineapples:*

*Pineapples, with their vibrant tropical flavour, bring a unique set of nutritional benefits to the table. Like bananas, pineapples are abundant in dietary fibre, aiding in digestion and promoting satiety. This fibre, combined with the fruit's natural sweetness, can help satisfy cravings for sugary snacks, making it an excellent choice for those looking to curb their sweet tooth while supporting their weight loss journey.*

*In addition to fibre, pineapples are a rich source of vitamin C, an antioxidant that supports immune function, collagen production, and skin health. They also contain bromelain, a mixture of enzymes that may help reduce inflammation, improve digestion, and accelerate wound healing.*

*Synergy of Nutrients: When combined in our "Banana Pineapple Drink," these two fruits create a synergistic blend of nutrients that work together to promote optimal health and weight management. The fibre content aids in digestion and curbing cravings, while the vitamins and minerals support immune function, energy metabolism, and overall well-being.*

*Understanding the nutritional components of bananas and pineapples allows us to appreciate the holistic benefits of our signature drink. In the following chapters, we will explore how these ingredients, along with other key additions, come together to create a potent elixir that not only tantalises the taste buds but also supercharges the body's fat-burning potential.*

# Chapter 3

## The Recipe for Success

*In this chapter, we unveil the simple yet potent recipe for the Banana Pineapple Drink, the ultimate weapon in your fat-blasting arsenal. With just a handful of ingredients and straightforward steps, you'll be on your way to sipping your way to a slimmer you.*

*Ingredients:*
*1 ripe banana*
*1 cup of fresh pineapple chunks*
*1 cup of coconut water*
*1 tablespoon of grated ginger*
*1 tablespoon of honey (optional, for added sweetness)*
*A squeeze of fresh lemon juice*

*Instructions:*

*1.Peel the banana and chop it into chunks.*

*2.Cut the fresh pineapple into small pieces, discarding the core.*

*3.In a blender, combine the banana chunks, pineapple chunks, grated ginger, coconut water, and honey (if using).*

*4.Squeeze in a generous amount of fresh lemon juice for a zesty kick.*

*5.Blend the ingredients until smooth and creamy.*

*6.Pour the mixture into a glass and garnish with a pineapple wedge or a sprig of mint for a touch of elegance.*

*7.Sip and enjoy the refreshing taste while knowing you're fueling your body with powerful fat-burning nutrients.*

*This simple yet effective recipe is the key to unlocking your fat-burning potential. With the natural sweetness of bananas and pineapples combined with the metabolism-boosting properties of ginger and lemon, you'll be well on your way to achieving your weight loss goals. So go ahead, whip up a batch of this delicious drink and toast to a healthier, slimmer you!*

# Chapter 4
## IncorporatingtheDrinkintoYour Routine

*Now that you have the recipe for the Banana Pineapple Drink that promises to burn fat like crazy, it's time to make it a seamless part of your daily routine. Whether you're a morning person, a gym enthusiast, or simply someone looking for a refreshing beverage, here are some tips and ideas to incorporate this powerful drink into your lifestyle for maximum effectiveness.*

### 1.Start Your Day Right with a Morning Smoothie:

*Kickstart your metabolism by enjoying the Banana Pineapple Drink as a breakfast smoothie. Blend it with some Greek yoghurt or almond milk for added creaminess and protein. This will not only provide you with a nutritious start to your day but also keep you feeling full and energised until your next meal.*

### 2.Pre-Workout Boost:

*Fuel your body with the right nutrients before hitting the gym. Sip on the Banana Pineapple Drink about 30 minutes before your workout session to give yourself a natural energy boost. The combination of banana and pineapple will provide you with carbohydrates for energy, while the fat-burning properties of the drink will help you power through your exercise routine.*

*3.Post-Workout Recovery:*

*After a strenuous workout, it's essential to replenish your body with the necessary nutrients to aid in recovery. The Banana Pineapple Drink can serve as an excellent post-workout refreshment. Its high potassium content from bananas helps restore electrolyte balance, while the bromelain in pineapple can help reduce inflammation and promote muscle recovery.*

*4.Midday Pick-Me-Up:*

*Beat the afternoon slump with a refreshing glass of the Banana Pineapple Drink. Instead of reaching for sugary snacks or caffeine, opt for this natural, fat-burning beverage to keep you alert and focused throughout the day. The vitamins and minerals present in the drink will provide you with sustained energy without the crash.*

*5.Evening Indulgence:*

*Wind down in the evening with a chilled glass of the Banana Pineapple Drink. Skip the calorie-laden desserts and opt for this guilt-free treat instead. Its natural sweetness will satisfy your cravings while its fat-burning properties will help support your weight loss goals even as you relax.*

*Incorporating the Banana Pineapple Drink into your daily routine is not only easy but also beneficial for your overall health and fitness goals. Whether you prefer it as a morning smoothie, a pre-workout boost, or an evening indulgence, this drink is sure to become a staple in your diet. Cheers to a healthier, slimmer you!*

# *Chapter 5*

# Testimonials and Success Stories

*Welcome to the chapter where real-life transformations unfold before your eyes. The Banana Pineapple Drink isn't just a refreshing beverage; it's a catalyst for change, a potion of possibilities. Let's dive into the inspiring journeys of those who have embraced this elixir and reaped its rewards.*

### 1. Sarah's Story:

*Sarah had struggled with her weight for years, trying every fad diet and trendy workout routine with little success. Frustrated and disheartened, she stumbled upon the Banana Pineapple Drink recipe and decided to give it a shot. Within weeks, she noticed a significant difference in her energy levels and a gradual but steady decline in her weight. With renewed confidence, Sarah embraced a healthier lifestyle, and today, she's proud to flaunt her toned physique.*

### 2. Mark's Testimony:

*For Mark, it wasn't just about shedding pounds; it was about reclaiming his life. Battling obesity and its associated health issues, he was on the verge of giving up hope. Then, he stumbled upon the Banana*

*Pineapple Drink and decided to commit to a daily regimen. The results were astonishing. Not only did he lose weight, but his cholesterol levels dropped, his blood pressure stabilised, and he felt more alive than ever before. Mark's journey serves as a beacon of hope for anyone facing similar struggles.*

### *3. Emily's Triumph:*

*Emily was tired of feeling sluggish and out of shape. Despite her best efforts, she couldn't seem to find the motivation to stick to a healthy routine. That is until she discovered the Banana Pineapple Drink. Not only did it kickstart her metabolism, but it also ignited a newfound passion for fitness. Armed with renewed vigour, Emily embraced a regular exercise routine and watched as the pounds melted away. Today, she's the epitome of vitality and serves as an inspiration to those around her.*

### *4. Jason's Journey:*

*Jason had always been sceptical of so-called "miracle cures" for weight loss. But when he stumbled upon the Banana Pineapple Drink, something resonated with him. He decided to give it a try, albeit with a healthy dose of scepticism. To his surprise, the results were undeniable. Not only did he lose weight, but he also felt more energised and focused throughout the day. Jason's transformation serves as a reminder that sometimes, the most extraordinary results come from the simplest of ingredients.*

*5. Maria's Miracle:*

*Maria had struggled with yo-yo dieting for years, bouncing between extremes in search of a quick fix. It wasn't until she discovered the Banana Pineapple Drink that she realised sustainable weight loss was within reach. Not only did the drink help her shed pounds, but it also curbed her cravings and stabilised her mood. Today, Maria enjoys a balanced lifestyle, free from the shackles of restrictive diets and endless cycles of deprivation.*

*These testimonials and success stories are just a glimpse into the transformative power of the Banana Pineapple Drink. Whether you're looking to shed stubborn pounds, boost your energy levels, or simply reclaim your vitality, this potent elixir holds the key to unlocking your full potential. Are you ready to join the ranks of the transformed?*

# Chapter 6
## Frequently Asked Questions

In this chapter, we address some of the most commonly asked questions about the Banana Pineapple Drink, ensuring that any lingering doubts or concerns are thoroughly answered.

Question:

Is the Banana Pineapple Drink safe for diabetics?

Answer:

Yes, the Banana Pineapple Drink is safe for diabetics when consumed in moderation. Both bananas and pineapples have a moderate glycemic index, meaning they won't cause a rapid spike in blood sugar levels when consumed. However, it's always wise for individuals with diabetes to monitor their carbohydrate intake and consult with a healthcare professional before incorporating any new foods or drinks into their diet.

Question:

*Can I consume the Banana Pineapple Drink if I'm trying to lose weight?*

*Answer:*

*Absolutely! The Banana Pineapple Drink can be a great addition to a weight loss plan. It's low in calories and contains ingredients like bananas and pineapples, which are rich in fibre and water, helping you feel full and satisfied for longer periods. Plus, the metabolism-boosting properties of the ingredients may aid in fat burning.*

*Question:*

*Is the Banana Pineapple Drink suitable for vegetarians/vegans?*

*Answer:*

*Yes, the Banana Pineapple Drink is completely plant-based and suitable for vegetarians and vegans. It contains no animal products or by-products, making it a perfect choice for those following a plant-based lifestyle.*

*Question:*

*Can I make substitutions or additions to the Banana Pineapple Drink recipe?*

*Answer:*

*Absolutely! While the recipe provided in this book is a delicious and effective combination for burning fat, feel free to customise it to suit your taste preferences or dietary needs. You can experiment with different fruits, such as adding berries or mango, or incorporating ingredients like spinach or kale for an extra nutritional boost.*

*Question:*

*How often should I drink the Banana Pineapple Drink to see results?*

*Answer:*

*For optimal results, we recommend incorporating the Banana Pineapple Drink into your daily routine as part of a balanced diet and regular exercise regimen. However, individual results may vary, so listen to your body and adjust the frequency of consumption based on your goals and how your body responds.By addressing these frequently asked questions, we hope to provide clarity and reassurance to readers interested in incorporating the Banana Pineapple Drink into their lifestyle. Remember, always consult with a healthcare professional before making any significant changes to your diet or exercise routine.*

# Chapter 7

## Conclusion - Cheers to a Healthier You!

*Congratulations on reaching the end of this journey towards a healthier lifestyle! Throughout this book, we've explored the incredible benefits of the Banana Pineapple Drink and how it can aid in burning fat like crazy while boosting your overall well-being. Now, as we wrap up our discussion, let's recap some of the key takeaways and toast to your success!*

*First and foremost, the Banana Pineapple Drink is a powerhouse of nutrition. Packed with vitamins, minerals, and antioxidants, it provides your body with essential nutrients to support overall health and vitality. By incorporating this delicious beverage into your daily routine, you're giving your body the fuel it needs to thrive.*

*One of the most remarkable benefits of the Banana Pineapple Drink is its ability to aid in fat loss. Thanks to its metabolism-boosting ingredients and low-calorie content, it can help you shed those extra pounds and achieve your weight loss goals more effectively. Plus, its natural sweetness satisfies cravings without adding unnecessary calories, making it a guilt-free indulgence.*

*But the benefits don't stop there. The Banana Pineapple Drink also supports digestion, promotes hydration, and boosts energy levels, helping you feel your best both inside and out. Whether you're looking to slim down, improve your overall health, or simply enjoy a refreshing beverage, this drink is sure to become a staple in your daily routine.*

*As you embark on your fat-loss journey, remember to stay consistent and patient. Rome wasn't built in a day, and neither is a healthier body. By making small, sustainable changes to your diet and lifestyle, and incorporating the Banana Pineapple Drink into your routine, you'll be well on your way to achieving the results you desire.*

*So here's to you and your commitment to a healthier, happier you! Cheers to making positive changes, embracing a balanced lifestyle, and enjoying the journey every step of the way. With the Banana Pineapple Drink by your side, the possibilities are endless. Here's to a brighter, healthier future - bottoms up!*

# Chapter 8